NATURAL WAYS TO TREAT TYPE 2

DIABETES

Copyright 2017

Natural Ways to Treat Type 2 Diabetes

Table of Contents

Introduction

Type 2 Diabetes

Statistics of Type 2 Diabetes

Diagnosis of Type 2 Diabetes

Natural Ways to Treat Type 2 Diabetes

Ways to Reduce Type 2 Diabetes

Summary

APPENDIX A

Additional Resources

Natural Ways to Treat Type 2 Diabetes

DISCLAIMER: this book is not intended to be construed as health advice. Please consult a medical doctor / physician if you have any ailments.

To My Family and Friends

Introduction

This book is intended to give information regarding type 2 diabetes. Leaving type 2 diabetes untreated can lead to serious health consequences. This book discusses some of the tests and ways that type 2 diabetes is diagnosed.

Also discussed are some of the lifestyle behaviors that cause type 2

Natural Ways to Treat Type 2 Diabetes

diabetes. This book also gives some

information about some lifestyle changes

that one can undergo to treat this condition.

Type 2 Diabetes

Type 2 diabetes is a condition in which ones body cannot process or make enough insulin properly. This causes the blood glucose sugar levels in the blood to rise. Not treating type 2 diabetes can lead to serious health consequences such as amputation and death.

The American Diabetes Association (ADA) defines type 2 diabetes as 'a problem with your body that 'causes blood glucose

Natural Ways to Treat Type 2 Diabetes

(sugar) levels to rise higher than normal.'
This is also called hyperglycemia.

Type 2 diabetes is the most common
form of diabetes and will only be addressed
in this book; that is, type 1 diabetes will not
be addressed in this book. As mentioned, if
one has type 2 diabetes, one's body does not
use insulin properly. This is called insulin
resistance.

When one's body works normally, the
pancreas makes extra insulin when one's
blood glucose sugar rises. Insulin moves
blood glucose sugar out of the blood and

Natural Ways to Treat Type 2 Diabetes

into cells. However, over time if the

pancreas isn't able to make enough insulin or

keep up with insulin production of one's

blood glucose at normal levels, pre-diabetes,

or worse, type 2 diabetes sets in.

Statistics of Type 2 Diabetes

One can argue that type 2 diabetes has become an epidemic. Millions of people throughout the world have or had type 2 diabetes. According to the American Diabetes Association, in 2015, 30.3 million Americans, or 9.4% of the population, had type 2 diabetes. Of that amount, approximately 1.25 million American children and adults have type 1 diabetes. Of the 30.3 million Americans with diabetes, 23.1 million were diagnosed and 7.2 million were undiagnosed. With that said, early detection of type 2 diabetes is critical to prevention.

Diabetes is very prevalent among senior citizens. The percentage of Americans with type 2 diabetes age sixty-five (65) and older remains high, at 25.2%, or twelve (12) million seniors (diagnosed and undiagnosed).

There are 1.5 million new cases of Americans that are newly diagnosed with diabetes every year. In 2015, 84.1 million

Natural Ways to Treat Type 2 Diabetes

Americans age eighteen (18) and older had pre-diabetes. Again these statistics underscore the argument that type 2 diabetes is an epidemic.

Diabetes remains one of the largest killing diseases. According to the American Diabetes Association, diabetes was responsible for being the seventh (7th) leading cause of death in the United States. In 2015, 79,535 death certificates listed type 2 diabetes as the underlying cause of death, and a total of 252,806 death certificates listed diabetes as an underlying or

contributing cause of death.

Diabetes can be found in all ethnic races,

it does not discriminate. The following

shows the prevalence of type 2 diabetes by

race:

7.4% of non-Hispanic whites

8.0% of Asian Americans

12.1% of Hispanics

12.7% of non-Hispanic blacks

15.1% of American Indians/Alaskan Native Indians

(source: American Diabetes Association)

Diabetes may be underreported as a cause of death. Studies have found that only about thirty-five (35%) to forty percent (40%) of people with diabetes who died had diabetes listed anywhere on the death certificate. About ten (10%) to fifteen (15%) percent of people had it listed as the underlying cause of death. (source:

American Diabetes Association).

Natural Ways to Treat Type 2 Diabetes

Diagnosis of Type 2 Diabetes

It is critical that one get tested for

diabetes. A medical doctor / physician can

administer a blood test to check one's blood

glucose sugar level. The test checks the

A1C and eAG levels in the blood.

The A1C and eAG test gives an

overall picture of one's average blood

glucose (blood sugar) control for the past

two to three months. One will have to make

two or three visits to the doctor's office to

determine the baseline of the A1C and eAG levels.

If the test levels are high there are a few ways to get the A1C and eAG levels reduced. Some of the ways are through simple modifications to one's lifestyle, as explained in the next three sections of the book.

Natural Ways to Treat Type 2 Diabetes

Ways to Reduce Type Diabetes

There are several dietary changes that one can make to reduce blood glucose / sugar levels. The first way is to eliminate refined white sugars. Refined white sugars can be found in candy, ice cream, sodas, fruit juices and packaged food products.

It is hard to not come across a product that doesn't not have added sugar in it. Processed foods such as cookies, cereal and crackers are fortified and loaded with added sugar. So one way to check to see if there is any sugar in packaged food products is to

read the labels on the products that you are

shopping for.

REDUCING STARCHES

Another way to reduce type 2 diabetes

is to reduce white starches. Although this

might not be as obvious as sugar, white

starches can easily be converted into sugar

and greatly increase blood glucose sugar

levels. White starches can be found in the

following foods:

White breads,

White potatoes

White rice.

Refined white flour products such as

pasta and baked goods

NON-STARCHY VEGETABLES

While reducing or eliminating white sugar and white starches is suggested, there are some alternative foods to substitute such as non-starchy vegetables. Some common non-starchy vegetable food alternatives are as follows:

Amaranth or Chinese spinach

Artichoke

Artichoke hearts

Asparagus

Baby corn

Bamboo shoots

Beans (green, wax, Italian)

Bean sprouts

Beets

Brussels sprouts

Broccoli

Cabbage (green, bok choy, Chinese)

Carrots

Cauliflower

Celery

Chayote

Coleslaw (packaged, no dressing)

Cucumber

Daikon

Eggplant

Greens (collard, kale, mustard, turnip)

Hearts of palm

Jicama

Kohlrabi

Leeks

Mushrooms

Okra

Onions

Pea pods

Peppers

Radishes

Rutabaga

Salad greens (chicory, endive, escarole, lettuce, romaine, spinach, arugula, radicchio, watercress)

Sprouts

Squash (cushaw, summer, crookneck, spaghetti, zucchini)

Sugar snap peas

Swiss chard

Tomato

Turnips

Water chestnuts

Yard-long beans

Some other foods suggested are:

Whole grains, oatmeal, quinoa, millet, or amaranth

Brown Rice

Baked sweet potato

Items made with whole grains and zero

(or very little) added sugar

WORST CHOICES OF FOOD FOR

TYPE 2 DIABETICS

In addition to sugars and white starches, there are several other foods that can contribute to type 2 diabetes. Below is a list of some of the worst choices of foods to consume for pre-diabetics and type 2 diabetics.

Processed grains, such as white rice or white flour

Natural Ways to Treat Type 2 Diabetes

Cereals with little whole grains and lots of sugar

White bread

French fries

Fried / white-flour tortillas

Natural Ways to Treat Type 2 Diabetes

A summary of foods to avoid can be found in Appendix A of this book.

One should also stop eating processed foods and substituting them for whole foods such as fruits, vegetables, herbs and lean meats, preferably organic in nature as organic food is not treated with pesticides, chemicals and genetically modified organisms (GMOs). Scientists, consumer and environmental groups have cited many health and environmental risks with foods containing GMOs. Leave the processed white flour-based products, especially the ones with added sugar, on the shelves or use

them only for special occasion treats.

SUGGESTED AMOUNT OF DIETARY

SUGAR INTAKE

One can eliminated sugar from their diet, but this can be a very difficult and tedious process to do. In many cases, eliminating refined, white sugar and white starches is next to impossible to do, so one alternative is to reduce the consumption of sugar to certain levels per meal, per day.

Upon the medical advice from my doctor, my doctor suggested that I consume or reduce my levels of sugar. She suggested

Natural Ways to Treat Type 2 Diabetes

that I portion my meals to no more than ten

(10) grams of sugar per meal. By doing this,

no more than thirty (30) grams of sugar is to

be consumed per day.

<u>Summary</u>

As mentioned, type 2 diabetes is very prevalent across society and one can argue that it has become an epidemic. Millions of people throughout the world have or had type 2 diabetes. As explained in this book, different foods can trigger type 2 diabetes.

Getting tested by your doctor is crucial for diagnosing diabetes. Ensuring that a medical doctor administers the correct test mentioned in this book will allow one to get a head start on treating type 2 diabetes if diagnosed.

Most importantly, avoid or restrict refined sugar and white starches such as refined flour, white bread, white potatoes and white rice. Knowledge and prevention is the key to treating type 2 diabetes.

APPENDIX A

List of Foods that a Type 2 Diabetic

Should Avoid

Refined, white sugars found in:

Candy

Cakes

Soda, pop

Ice Cream

Fruit Juices

White Starches such as:

White Bread

White Potatoes

White Rice

Refined Flour products found in pasta

and baked goods such as cookies and cakes

DISCLAIMER: this book is not intended to be construed as health advice. Please consult a physician if you have any ailments.

.

ADDITIONAL RESOURCES

Natural Ways to Treat Type 2 Diabetes

OTHER SUGGESTED BOOKS LINKS

(available in Kindle too!)

Herb and Spices and their Antioxidant

Properties

http://amzn.to/2jRqLuk

Growing Vegetables, Fruits and Herbs in the

Middle-Atlantic Region of the United States

http://amzn.to/2jMvCge

Deep Nutrition: Herbs and Spices:

Antioxidant Properties, Health and Healing

(includes Cloves and Cinnamon)

http://amzn.to/2iFKnOq

Nutrition: Growing Vegetables, Fruits and

Herbs in the Middle Atlantic Region of the

United States: Growing Fruits and Planting

Vegetables Book

http://amzn.to/2ze5KN4

AUTHOR'S YOUTUBE CHANNELS

https://www.youtube.com/channel/UCq7u

NSjONd6E8tsvErAHqNQ

https://www.youtube.com/channel/UC9xo

Y04t1q4whrjPjf2b0Uw

Natural Ways to Treat Type 2 Diabetes

AUTHOR'S BLOGS

https://thestockmarketinvestorblog.blogs

pot.com

https://thestockpicker2010.blogspot.com

https://stockmarketinvestorblog.blogspot.

com

https://thestockpickingblog.blogspot.com

https://thevalueinvestorblog.blogspot.com

https://personalfinancetimes.blogspot.com

https://theeconomicanalyst.blogspot.com

https://mymoneymakingtipsblog.blogspot.com

https://weightlossdecrease.blogspot.com

AUTHOR'S FACEBOOK PAGE

https://facebook.com/stock.trader.39

TWITTER

@Jrlvt

LINKS TO SUPPORT THE AUTHOR'S

WORK

SHOP AT THE AMAZON LINK

BELOW TO SUPPORT AUTHOR'S

WORK:

https://amzn.to/2gRrd9W

MAKE A PAYPAL CONTRIBUTION

TO SUPPORT AUTHOR'S WORK:

https://paypal.me/JamesLynd

PERFECT THREADS CLOTHING

COMPANY

Check out the author's clothing company at the link below, you can create your very own clothing / shirts; once inside the link, just click on the "CREATE' link to get started:

https://shop.spreadshirt.com/PerfectThreads

OTHER INFORMATION

The author has a Master of Business Administration degree with a concentration in Finance from the University of Baltimore and a Bachelor of Science Degree from Virginia Tech. In addition to having interests in money, investing and wealth, the author has interests in building businesses, e-commerce, sports, travel and organic gardening.

NOTES SECTION

NOTES SECTION

Natural Ways to Treat Type 2 Diabetes

END

Natural Ways to Treat Type 2 Diabetes

www.ingramcontent.com/pod-product-compliance
Lightning Source LLC
Chambersburg PA
CBHW030036230526
45472CB00002B/537